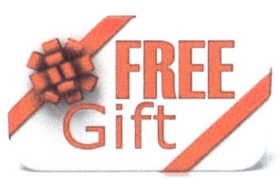

Want Priority Access to FREE eBooks Additional Materials for this Book?

As we release NEW eBooks, we offer them for FREE for a limited time. You will be the FIRST one to know when they are FREE. Join 1000's of insiders who are getting access to FREE Kindle book promotions weekly.

Click HERE for FREE additional material and FREE eBooks-
www.rictamilypublishing.com

Table of Contents

Introduction to Oil Pulling

What are you going to do if someone will ask you to wash your mouth with oil? Honestly, it sounds disgusting and greasy so I'm quite not interested to do that to my very own mouth because I feed myself through it and who wants to feel slime all over his or her mouth? But when I learned about a therapy which uses oil to cure diseases and oral problems, I admit I became a little bit fascinated until I discovered all the benefits it could provide. Let me tell you that this kind of therapy requires you to be more patient and responsible.

I read about a story of an Indian whose teeth were rattling which causes extreme pain through is head and jaw. The dentist told him that the rot was too deep, so he needs extraction. He was so afraid to undergo the extraction until six months later; his friend came to him and said that he knew about this alternative therapist who prescribes sunflower oil as mouthwash. No extraction and all 32 teeth intact!

If you have no idea about what oil therapy is about, join us as we discover the health benefits of oil pulling together.

The brainchild of this wonderful therapy is Dr. F Karach who suggests rinsing the gums and the teeth very carefully with a tablespoon of any vegetable oil. A person must do it really slowly for good 15 to 20 minutes three times a day with an empty stomach.

At first, the oil hisses viciously inside your mouth, but as the body's digestive juices dilute it, it turns out to be thin and white like milk in color then it should spit out right after and brush the teeth. Dr. Karach studied the gargled oil under a 600 magnification microscope and he discovered live organisms bathing in it. He warns that it is really poisonous, so you should never swallow it. The said poisons are the bacteria-embryos, which, if not eradicated could cause viruses and infections. Seemingly, Dr. Karach healed his own chronic blood illness and arthritis that he's been battling with for 15 years.

The very first sign of progress is when the teeth become whiter and firm. Others are feeling more relaxed on waking up, fresh, the dark pouches under the eyes disappears, unexplainable energy and full appetite, deep sleep and better memory.

Dr. Karach insists that by just gargling vegetable oil, anything under the sun like organ-disorders, menstrual problems, skin-diseases and paralysis in the human anatomy can be healed. You can do it even when you have a fever and added that it only takes two days to a year to cure a disease. If this sounds overwhelming, he told the cancer specialist to try it for themselves.

Conferring to life science, the tongue is charted by organ positions and that is, each section of the tongue is linked to the different organs of the body, such as the lungs, liver, kidney, spleen, heart, stomach, colon, small intestines, spine and pancreas. Therefore an oil massage in the mouth arouses and calms the key meridians where the taste encounters the organ.

Chapter 1

What is Oil Pulling?

Oil pulling is pretty much a simple process, completely harmless and totally inexpensive, unlike the common medical treatments available in the market. The only thing you need is a spoonful of vegetable oil daily. Yes, I am serious that this medication is cheaper than your daily vitamins. But let me tell you a secret, this is probably one of the most powerful types of therapy. Please tell as many as you can that I told you that.

One amazing fact about oil pulling is its simplicity as it is made of natural remedies and won a lot of hearts of people around the globe. It is strongly believed that the most apparent result of oil pulling is under the oral health category. Gums are healthier and way lot pinker, the teeth become whiter and the breath also becomes fresher. Who doesn't want white teeth, pink gums and fresh breath? In this therapy, you don't need to spend more than$100 to get that! This alone makes doing this brilliant therapy worthy!

What's more extraordinary is that oil pulling also helps to cure other health problems. Oil pulling has the possibility to cure any disease or chronic condition. The results of the oil pulling therapy appealed bewilderment and hesitation concerning its effectiveness and legitimacy. It is really superb that the effects that are achieved are truly made under the harmless organic therapeutic method. This really simple method proves it likely is to be effective to treat the most wide-ranging diseases. In some cases, medications are being set aside because of this because most medicines have side effects while the organic way gives you a natural healing process so you can enjoy and not worry about your liver, your palpitating heart and sleeping problems.

The thrilling element of the oil pulling curing method is its plainness. It contains of swishing or drawing cold-pressed oil into the mouth. The healing procedure is done by the human organism on its own. This is possible to heal tissues, cells and all organs all together, gets rid of the body's toxic waste without troubling the healthy microflora. A doctor in this field named Dr. Karach said that human beings only live half of their life span. A person could possibly live up to 140 to 150 years old under the healthy lifestyle.

Chapter 2

Oil Used in Oil Pulling

Dr. Karach recommends using sunflower oil, which also has alternative suggested oil, the sesame oil. We have different experiences with different oils so experimentation is the key. Trying different types of oil could also help to see what suits you best. You can try oil pulling in shorter or longer time, whatever makes you feel better. The only thing that separates a person from another person is the palatability. If you can't stand it, spit it out.

Sesame oil is a lot warmer rather than any other oils and can be gentler in detoxifying than other types of oil which are colder vigorous. It has a strong sesame taste, though, which is very familiar in terms of food taste for most of us. Sunflower oil has a lighter taste if you want that. Coconut oil is typical for most of us, too. It has, the calmer energy like the sesame oil so it's good for people who like to have a warmer constitution of heat. Some have described that coconut oil is more detoxifying which isn't that of a good thing because it is still best to get things cautiously and slowly.

Like what we have explained a number of times before, oil pulling cure and oil pulling method is extremely individual. With that said, the oil that is commonly used for this traditionally speaking is the sesame oil. If you are fine with the taste, you could go for that and appreciate how it goes.

Frequently Asked Questions: Oil Used in Oil Pulling

Q: Which oils should be avoided for oil pulling process?

Avoid all low quality oils that you wouldn't like to eat. Those contain canola oil, corn oil, soy oil, and cottonseed oil and those that go reeking very rapidly such as flax oil.

Q: Is it required to use cold-pressed, raw oil?

It is suggested that organic, raw, cold pressed oils with the life, vigor of the core ingredients in that oil are complete. Use the best value of oil you can get —untreated, cold-pressed, which does not contain chemical residues. If the only thing you see is refined oil, go for the sunflower oil or sesame oil, both of them will work efficiently.

Q: Is toasted oils allowed for oil pulling?

Do your best to avoid toasted oils because the high heat damages them.

Q: In most stores I only see expeller pressed oils, but never a cold pressed one. What else should I do?

Expeller pressed oil or cold pressed oil is just better quality oil that doesn't have chemical residues, and is healthier nutritionally. Refined oils are mostly high heated which harms the value to some degree, but still works fine for the prime purpose of oil pulling.

The exclusion process used for expeller pressed oils does make a definite quantity of heat, depending on the kind of seed or nut and how much pressure it takes to acquire the oil out of it. But this is really low compared to the high heatedprocess used for refined oils. Search for a brand of oil with unrefined, natural, organic sunflower oil or sesame oil.

Q: Can we add oil of oregano or other essential oils to the oil used in oil pulling?

Please do not add any oil to the oil you have designated for oil pulling. For example you chose sunflower oil, then stick to it and just use that type of oil. It is our contemporary day lifestyle that we are dying to add flavor to almost everything in life. Unfortunately, by following the stereotypes we end up messing with life's natural qualities.

Chapter 3

The Oil Pulling Method

Every morning that you wake up, before you put something inside your growling hungry stomach, take time to appreciate this therapy that could help you and make your body thank you after ten years.

Oil pulling is just a simple process. Take one spoonful of sunflower oil into the mouth but never swallow it! Move it slowly as swishing or rinsing and as Dr. Karach puts it like this, "sip, suck and pull through the teeth" for a good fifteen to twenty minutes. This process makes oil, concentrated and mixed with the saliva. Swishing triggers the enzymes and these enzymes eradicate toxins out of the blood. The oil should not and never be swallowed because it is poisonous and considered toxic. As the process goes on, the oil becomes thinner and white. If the color of the oil is still yellow, then it's not been pulled enough, but if it's already white, then you can spit it out and rinse the whole oral cavity and mouth carefully. You don't need special substance to clean things up because you can use the good old little fingers to clean it.

After this you can clean the sink and use antibacterial soap to finish it because the gargled material contains a lot of harmful bacteria and toxic bodily waste. It's really significant to know that through the oil swishing or an oil pulling process one's metabolism is strengthened. And guess what, this lead to improved and good health. One of the outstanding results of the oil pulling process is the noticeable whitening of the teeth, less bleeding of gums and clasping of loose teeth.

The oil swishing or oil pulling process is best done before meals to quicken its healing course. The process can be repeated thrice a day, but do not forget to do it before meals or with an unfilled stomach.

Here are some of the precautions while doing the oil pulling therapy:

- DO NOT SWALLOW. The gargled oil must be spat out.
- If you're allergic to a specific brand of oil, modify the brand or oil itself to a dissimilar kind of oil.
- Sesame and Sunflower oil has been found really effective in healing diseases. Others were not identified as well, so do not point fingers on oil pulling for performing it with other oils.

Oil Pulling: The Step-By-Step Process

Step #1

The very first thing you have to do as you wake up in the morning is not to eat nor drink, but instead on an empty stomach and before drinking any liquids including water, drizzle one spoonful of sesame or sunflower oil into your mouth. We do not commend doing this method at another time. Children could also do this process with less amount of oil on condition that they have control and preparation not to swallow the oil.

Step #2

You must swish the oil around your mouth without swallowing it, then start moving it round your mouth, then to your teeth as if you are gargling your favorite mouthwash. Do not tilt your head backwards because you might swallow it. You will feel that the oil starts getting watery as the saliva blends with it. Keep hissing, but if your jaw feels sore, then you're doing it wrong. Ease the jaw muscles and use the tongue to support and move the liquid inside your mouth.

There is no right or wrong way in swishing or pulling oil so you need not to focus on doing it right. You just have to do it in a natural way, as gentle as you could, but never vigorously, just relax and swish thoroughly for about 15 to 20 minutes. If you find it unbearable because it feels unpleasant, you can spit it out and do it again. If you're not used to it, it really feels nasty, but when you do it over and over again, you'll get used to it just like how you do brush your teeth.

When the oil has been soaked with the toxins it has eradicated, the color whitens, and the liquid becomes thinner, a milky consistency- depending on the type of oil used. Each time you pull the oil, it can take the dissimilar amount of time to acquire to that point, so 20 minutes are the fine line however you can experiment with this.

If you spit it out prior 20 minutes, you have to start again. This procedure is to make the oil swish have an ample time in your mouth so that it turn into a white thick substance which is the hint of the process accomplishment.

Step #3

After all the swishing process, we are now heading to the last step which is spitting the oil out of the mouth. When you see that the color of the oil is white, you can spit it out already and rinse your mouth thoroughly with warm salt water. You can use the standard table salt, but this isn't that necessary. Salt water cleaning is helpful in terms of removing the micro bacteria and soothing any swelling and is proven to be effective in washing away the toxins which may be left out inside the mouth.

You can practice oil pulling every morning if you want to or not necessarily every day because this method is detoxifying which you might want to take a break from time to time. One direct benefit every person gets is cleaner mouth and whiter teeth. There is no rule regarding the frequency, but you can evaluate by your own experience.

You must know that oil pulling works better in the morning rather than any other time. Do not try to do this any time of the day. If for some reason it is totally not possible for you to do this in the morning, you can practice this on an empty stomach at any time of the day. Empty stomach simply means that the food is digested entirely, preferably over three to four hours after food intake but it still depends on what food you ate.

Chapter 4

Effects of Oil Pulling

The outcomes of this healing study has both fascinated and shocked a lot of people, which resulted in a more advanced research. The further research about oil therapy has now been carefully documented, particularly with regard to physiological comparisons amid individuals.

It is indeed surprising that through this natural healing method, a wide-ranging variety of symptoms have absolutely vanished without any side effects reported from the people who tried it for themselves. This simple technique makes it promising to completely cure such well known diseases which would usually be treated by an operation or by influential or potent drugs, which typically has significant side effects.

The simplicity of this medical system in which oil is churned back to the front of the mouth is due to the effect of stimulation which it has on the body's eliminatory system. Through this process, it is possible to cure individual cells, cell conglomerates such as complex tissues in the internal organs and lymph nodes simultaneously. This happens because the helpful microflora in the body is delivered with a vigorous continuum. Without the body's natural invasive element exhibited by the microflora, the typical pattern of human health inclines to lean en route for illness rather than wellness.

Dr. Karach expects that consistent application of this treatment by backing this process so that wellness is the overriding state of the human body and is possible to increase the normal human lifespan to roughly 150 years, double the present life probability.

He was also supported in this assessment by other associates in the world. By just doing this oil pulling treatment, it is always the result that sicknesses such as bronchitis, migraine headaches, arterio thrombosis, diseased teeth, and chronic blood disorders like leukemia, arthritis, neuro physiological paralysis, kidney disease, eczema, peritonitis, gastro enteritis, heart disease, meningitis, and women's hormonal conditions are utterly eradicated from the organism.

The advantage of Dr. Karach'sway is that the oil treatment heals the entire body in imperishability. In fatal diseases just like cancer or AIDS, and other chronic infections, this curing method has been exposed to successfully substitute all others. Dr. Karach has successfully cured a patient suffering from chronic leukemia with 15 years of severe treatment procedures behind him and a patient who was completely bedridden and has acute arthritis which was eradicated from his body in 3 days with no infection apparent.

Chapter 5

In Depth Discussion: Oral Health Benefits of Oil Pulling Method

One of the most cost effective ways to have whiter and stronger teeth is through the process of oil pulling. If the eyes are the window to one's soul, then the mouth is the window of one's body's health. Oral health can bargain tons of clues in regards to your overall health. Just so you know, our overall health is thoroughly connected to our oral health and hygiene more than we ever realize.

Your oral health is linked to many other health conditions beyond just the mouth itself. Often times, the first sign of infection shows up in your pretty little mouth. In some cases, swelling in the mouth like gum diseases that could cause problems in other areas of the body.

The Connection of Oral Health to One's Overall Health

Scientists from the 87th GSIADR (General Session of the International Association for Dental Research) stated new studies linking oral diseases with general illnesses. A frequent theme is the connection between periodontal or gum disease and newborn prematurity, stroke, or diabetes. Oil pulling consumers all over the globe is generous enough to give evidence that by doing oil pulling, they were receiving lots of benefits.

Your mouth is usually packed with bacteria. Typically you can have these bacteria in control with decent oral health care, such as brushing your teeth daily and do not forget to do the flossing. Saliva too is a key protection against bacteria and diseases. It has enzymes that abolish bacteria in different means. But dangerous bacteria can occasionally grow out of hand and lead to a serious gum infection called periodontitis.

When your gums are in good physical shape, bacteria in your mouth commonly don't enter your bloodstream. Still, gum disease may deliver bacteria a haven of entry into the bloodstream. Sometimes aggressive dental actions also can let bacteria to enter the bloodstream. And medicines or treatments that decrease saliva flow or disturb the normal equilibrium of bacteria in your mouth also might lead to oral fluctuations, making it stress-free from bacteria to go into your bloodstream. Some researchers consider that these bacteria and infection from your mouth are connected to further health problems in the rest of the body.

What You Can Possibly Do in Regards with Your Oral Health?

If you did not previously have enough motives to take good care of your mouth, gums and teeth, the relationship between your oral health and your overall health delivers even more. Resolve to exercise decent oral hygiene every day. By doing this, you are constructing an investment in your overall health, not just for now, but wait until your body say thank you in the future.

How Oil Pulling works with your Oral Health?

Many people ask, "How does oil can make such a miraculous healing?" What is the technical reason behind this? The oil pulling processes the oil and makes it work as an organic cleaner for oral health. Your body is the healer. Our body is set with the capability to heal from any infectious or deteriorating disease. Oil pulling eliminates disease-causing bacteria and toxins in the mouth that results in ill health. There is nothing surreptitious about it; it is like basic biology. Most of the bacteria that are part of oral biology in the mouth contain of a single cell with a fatty membrane which is the outer wall of the cell.

When you are undertaking oil pulling, fatty membranes of the bacteria are engrossed to the oil you are swishing or pulling. As you gargle the oil around your teeth and gums, the hiding bacteria under crevices will be sucked out of their hiding places and would mix with the oil. This is why you need to do oil pulling. Your saliva mixes with the oil and together they eradicate the toxins and help to increase the body's capacity to self-heal.

Oil pulling does wonders for eliminating all kinds of germs and decreasing the number of possibly harmful ones. But still research desires to be done to prove the effectiveness on shifting the percentage of good bacteria. Our suggestion is to retain healthy habits alongside with oil pulling therapy.

Chapter 6

Other Ailments That Can be cured through Oil Pulling

If you are curious on what other diseases that might be connected to our oral health, below are some examples of the conditions that you're might into or interested to know:

Pregnancy and Premature Birth

One of the main reasons why a pregnant woman should take care of her body, most especially what she eats and her oral health is because gum diseases have previously been linked to premature birth. If you want your baby safe, do the right thing as well.

Heart Diseases

Numerous types of heart disease relate to oral health, according to research. The said heart problems include stroke and clogged arteries. In some research, oral health seems to be connected to different cardiovascular diseases.

Diabetes

Another common disease nowadays is diabetes, but little did we know that is upsurges the possibility of different oral health problems and included in the list are dry mouth, gum disease, cavities, tooth loss and numerous types of oral infections. Contrariwise, our poor health care can be soon transformed to diabetes, which is a lot harder to control. Infections could cause the blood sugar to rise and we'll need more insulin to take a hand on it.

Osteoporosis

Just so you know, teeth are considered bones so yes, the major stages of bone problems and loss could show up in your teeth. Why? Because it has a direct contact of whatever you eat. These may generate a condition where the bone supporting your teeth is getting more and more vulnerable because of the infectious damage. Your dentist could possibly be able to spot this through repetitive checkups and X-rays but if it gets worse, you have to do something about it. ASAP.

HIV/AIDS

HIV or AIDS is one of the common diseases that is connected to oral health problems. Symptoms are ulcers, having dry mouth, and sore mucosal lesions. Mouth problems are caused by bacterial, viral or fungal infections and in some cases, severe gum contamination is one of the main symptoms of AIDS. This will sound nasty, but you'll soon grow white spots and unusual lesions in your mouth or on your tongue.

Other Conditions

Most of the diseases exist in your mouth first before you know whatever is going wrong all over the body. Such diseases include cancers, eating disorders, syphilis, substance abuse and gonorrhea.

Chapter 7

Practices to Maintain a Healthy Lifestyle

Our body is made out of trillions of cells, but as human beings, our naked eyes are not that gifted to have a look of that. We need a microscope to be able to accomplish that. Have you ever asked yourself, "What can this cell do? How can this cell affect my body?" Always remember that all the chemical makeup and changes that takes place in our system can only be done through cells. Starting from our food intake to the water drain down to the air we breathe has a big contribution to our cell's growth. In fact, we do all these things for the sake of our cells to live. The air we inhale goes straight to our lungs, then joins the blood until it reaches to the cells which help in the manufacturing of energy to all the cells of the body.

Likewise, the water we take reaches the cells carefully by the blood and stomach. After the food we ate has been digested, it feels inside the bloodstream and will be carried into the cells. The food we eat helps renew the cells and produce energy for our body. If we delay our meals, we're going to feel weak instantly so it's really important to eat on time and take care of what food reaches the body.

There are three things that a human being must always remember.

1. What food should a normal person eat?
2. How much exercise a person needs to totally eradicate the toxins inside the body?
3. How much rest is needed to regain the energy lost?

Obviously, human beings need to eat and rest because if we don't, we are all going to die. Only we are acting pretty ignorant on how to maintain the right partitions. We eat what we want, do whatever we want to do and sleep whenever we want to. Seriously, do you think you're doing it right? A big NO.

God planted all these vegetables and fruits to be consumed and not all to serve as a design for your salad. You have to eat it and not stare at it. If we consume them the way they are opting to, the problem is over. And it is indeed true that if we eat prior the sun goes down, we'll have enough time for our food to be digested and the toxins will be eradicated first thing in the morning. I swear by that!

Chapter 8

Oil Pulling as Replacement to Medicines

Not because there are substitutes and therapies, we can forget about taking care of our body. What we do is shifting our bodies to our lifestyle, but we are not providing what it truly needs and requires. For example, we don't drink 8 glasses or more of water. We eat thoughtlessly without thinking if what we're eating is good for us and we eat like there's not tomorrow, which is the reason why we aren't able to breathe properly. We don't pay in consideration of our body's natural rhythms.

Due to consistent bad habits, our body turns out to be extremely vulnerable to diseases. Now we can detect and cure it through science. But the chaos only begins there. The catastrophe is that science cannot detect everything. They allot medicines for such illnesses, but they do not take into consideration man's life. Doctors tell us to be lifelong enthusiasts of medicine and yes, we shadow them blindly. But our body remains to suffer year after year. There is, on the other hand, a way out to free us of these diseases. The perfect alternative to make our body accustomed of habits is to adjust our ways to suit our bodies. It is our body so we have to love our own.

This is the lone solution. We have no further option. If we don't revolutionize our lifestyle, we cannot set an end to our cruel health. Let us set aside our bad habits and lifestyle. Let us keep an eye on the new routine that ensemble the necessities of the body and to make it clean and disease-free.

The body has the ability to heal itself in a step by step process through a new food routine. Thus the medicine intake can be abridged gradually. One day will come that medicines are not going to be essential to you at all.

Chapter 9

Frequently Asked Questions: Oil Pulling

Q: Who are allowed to do the oil pulling therapy?

Everyone who is above five years of age can do oil pulling.

Q: What is the best time to do oil pulling?

The best time to do oil pulling is in the morning before any meals or on an empty stomach.

Q: Is there a time gap after doing the oil pulling therapy?

Rinse your mouth thoroughly after oil pulling and then you can eat and drink. No time gap is required.

Q: Can we multitask while doing oil therapy?

No. It is advised to do it gently and carefully.

Q: Are there differences in methods of oil pulling to cure different diseases such as chronic and acute?

Acute illnesses can be cured in two to four days following the steps mentioned in other chapters while chronically requires more time. One year or depending on your habits, kind of disease, age, and present general health.

Q: How long will it take to cure a specific disease?

It depends on the factors I mentioned in the question above. If you have a good habit and lifestyle, then it'll be easier.

Q: Are there side effects or reactions and can medicines still be used?

Mostly, there are no reactions and the curing is smooth. If you drink medicines, you can slowly decrease its intake as you find progress on the oil pulling therapy. OP fully eradicates toxins from your body. This therapy cannot totally cure your chronic disease, but can reduce the side effects of the chemical drugs you take.

Q: What if I don't want to do oil pulling, what are the other ways to heal my gum disease and protect my oral health?

Well, aside from brushing your teeth, flossing can be useful, but you must take note that it can also make matters worse as you shove the floss into the gum. You have to floss really gently. An oral irrigator like Waterpik is recommended. The warm water, salt rinsing is also comforting to help heal inflammations and infections. You should know that it is very essential for gums to be swollen from time to time. The teeth and gums are the reflection of what's going on inside the body.

Most often the dentists will recommend to get gum surgery because they all think their patients are not interested to know how to take care of themselves at home and on the other hand, the patients are not meticulous of the other techniques they could do. But if you work on your food and lifestyle, the gum inflammations will be resolved in no time.

Chapter 10

Frequently Asked Questions: Oil Pulling Method

Q: Am I required to brush my teeth before I do oil pulling?

No, there's no need to. Brushing your teeth is only essential after you have done the oil pulling process because you have to clean the mouth properly. Toxins are eradicated so it's important to rinse it thoroughly. You don't want bacteria floating inside your mouth.

Q: How long should I swish before the oil turns white? 5, 10 or 20 minutes?

So far, there is no rule for that because the different oils perform differently so stop paying attention to it. You have to do oil pulling 20 minutes max and you shall notice that the oil will turn white.

Q: Is it normal if I was only able to swish for less than 20 mins?

It is common to many people actually. Well, if you cannot take it for 20 minutes long, you can swish again. But you have to really try your best to get to the point because you will be amazed at how quickly you can get used to it.

Q: I really can't help swallowing the oil. Is it dangerous?

It's okay to swallow a little if you really can't prevent it, but remember, what you are trying to eradicate are toxins so you really need to pull it out of the body. When you feel that you're about to swallow it, spit it out and start over again.

Q: I could only withstand oil pulling for a few minutes because I get tired easily. Why?

Maybe you are doing it wrong. You have to just relax and do it carefully. Swish in a more relaxed way and soon enough you'll get used to it.

Q: Why do I need to do the oil pulling process on an empty stomach?

First of all, it could help you not to feel full if you get a little nauseous from the oil pulling process. Second, the cleansing effect is a little intimidating. Eating light will not be a problem so just judge how you feel. If you can oil pull in the morning with an empty stomach, then we're good.

Conclusion

Thank you for downloading this book!

I hope this book was able to help you to learn the benefits of oil pulling.

The next step is to practice what you've learned.

Finally, if you enjoyed this book, please take the time to share your thoughts and post a review on Amazon. It'd be greatly appreciated!

Thank you and good luck!

Review Link

If you enjoyed this book, we would really appreciate it if you could leave us a positive REVIEW?

P.S. **You can CLICK HERE to go directly to the book page** and leave your review and/or purchase our other books above. Alternatively, you can copy and paste this address into your browser --- http://amzn.to/1wCj3OE

Preview of "Paleo and Grain-Free Diet for Beginners"

Cookbook Recipes Using a Slow Cooker for Weight Loss

Chapter 1

Paleo Diet: Going Back to the Basics

In the past few years, the Paleo diet has become extremely popular. The Paleo diet is the eating regimen that was followed by our Paleolithic ancestors. It is a diet human beings evolved with. This diet follows the dietetic restrictions of our prehistoric ancestors, particularly the hunter-gatherer of old times. It is designed to replicate their nutritional habits; that is why it also goes by the name caveman's diet, the hunter-gatherer diet, and the Stone Age diet. It is based on the principle that human beings can attain better health and ideal weight by eating food high in fiber and protein, and by avoiding carbohydrates, sugar, dairy, grains and processed foods. Unlike the modern day fad diets, Paleo diet does not encourage periodic starvation and removal of solid food. It simply promotes good health and healthy weight loss through eating good food.

Introduced by gastroenterologist; Dr. Walter L. Voegtlin, who successfully treated gastric conditions of his patients, Paleo diet is now becoming popular among those who want to lose weight while staying healthy and disease free. Paleo is the healthiest way to eat as it is the only nutritional approach that goes with human genetics to help them stay energetic, strong and lean. It has been proved that the modern diet patterns we follow today is filled with refined foods, sugar, and Trans fats, which is the root of many degenerative diseases such as depression, cancer, obesity and heart disease.

Foundation for a Better Health

The main focus of this diet is to eat food that is closer to its natural state, hence, un-complicate your food to un-complicate your health; it is more of a lifestyle. The majority of the food suggested in this diet is organic, grass fed meat, seafood, nuts, eggs, fresh vegetables, fruits and healthy fats. Foods such as grains, legumes, refined and processed foods, dairy, salt, alcohol and refined sugar are prohibited. There are clear instructions of what to eat and what to avoid.

The basic structure of the Paleo diet comprises of the following:

Lean Proteins

Lean proteins develop strong muscles, healthy bones and better immune functions. Proteins also make a person feel satisfied over a long time period. Paleo diet suggests grass-fed meat and poultry to be a part of your Paleo plate, but it must not be processed.

Fruits and Vegetables

These are rich in antioxidants, minerals, vitamins and phytonutrients. The fruits allowed in Paleo diet include all kinds of berries, citrus fruits, apples, peaches, plums, cherries and nectarines. As a rule, a person on Paleo diet should eat 2/3 vegetables, fresh fruit of his choice, and 1/3 meat and fat for each meal (breakfast, lunch and dinner).

Healthy Fats from Nuts and Seeds

All nuts are allowed in the Paleo diet as they are a good source of healthy fats, except for peanuts; these are legumes. Another source of healthy fats includes olives, avocados, coconut oil and other cold pressed oils. Fish is also considered a paleo food and contains omega 3 fatty acids such as salmon, tuna and mackerel. Mustard oil is allowed as it is without additives.

Beverages

Beverages include pure juice from fruits and vegetables; unsweetened and must be taken in moderation. Water is the primary beverage, no sodas, fizzy drinks and diet drinks are allowed. Tea and coffee are acceptable if lightened with almond milk and not dairy milk.

Only the inflammatory, artificial, chemically processed food with unhealthy vegetable oils along with whole grains are not allowed in the Paleo diet as their carbohydrate content easily gets dissolved and spike the insulin level, which in turn prevents the fat from burning.

Benefits of Paleo Diet

There are many long term health benefits of living the Paleo way. If followed properly, it provides a wide array of health benefits along with protecting the body from many diseases. A few are listed below.

- Sustainable/feasible weight loss and fat burning.
- Improved/enhanced energy levels throughout the day.
- Reduced allergies.
- Stable/controlled blood sugar and blood pressure.
- Burning off stored fat.
- Improved/better heart and digestive health.
- Better/maximize immune system.
- Improved skin.
- Better glucose intolerance.
- Better management in appetite.

Overall, Paleo diet is rich in macro and micro nutrients, and most of the people have reported better mood, better energy and reduction in chronic problems after following the Paleo diet.

Weight Loss with Paleo Diet

Although, there are many diets out there that emphasize upon cutting down meat and strict calorie counting, Paleo diet is the one that gives you freedom from counting calories and let you eat the food that your body is designed to consume. The only concern is to avoid the modern food that the body can't digest effectively.

It is an excellent way to lose weight since this diet is rich in healthy fats and proteins and free from sugar and starches. Through this diet, you can boost your metabolism, have healthy and better digestion, regulate/control fat storing hormones and reduce hunger and starving. Through mainstream diets, people lose weight only temporarily at the cost of good health. They deprive their body of adequate proteins and fats. Unlike other diets, Paleo diet won't harm your metabolism or reduce any muscle mass, rather you can lose weight permanently without starving your stomach. The Paleo diet is more effective than others because:

- Low-glycemic carbs from plant sources reduce cravings and increase energy levels.
- Protein contributes majorly in building lean muscle and burn fat faster by slowing appetite.
- Omega-3 fatty acids and other healthy fats keep the level of blood sugar normal, reduce fatigue and help in burning the stored fat.
- Vitamin C consumed from vegetables and fruits boost the metabolism.

You might question that how a diet so rich in nutrients can help in weight management? This is because of the fiber component in its food, which is soluble and insoluble fiber. Soluble fiber when dissolved in water, becomes a gel like substance, traps bad cholesterol and slows down the digestion to maintain the feeling of fullness to prevent overeating. Whereas, the insoluble fibers help in better bowel movement by pushing the content out of the body smoothly and prevent constipation, which is a common problem among those trying to lose weight on unhealthy diets. It is not a fat free diet, but it is a bad-fat free diet.

So, Paleo diet is about working with your body and not against it, and hence, enhancing it to burn extra fat effectively and efficiently.

The following chapters include delicious slow cooker Paleo recipes that you can eat to burn those extra pounds. The benefit of Paleo food along with weight loss is the delicious taste and better health. Now, you don't have to eat tasteless and bland food to lose weight. One of the benefits of using a slow cooker is that it is fuss free, nutritious, and requires less to no supervision. Put the food in and go on with your regular daily activities, and come home to a delicious cooked meal. Slow cookers are best to put the most flavors in the foods. They are so easy to use that a beginner can confidently make delicious meals with them. Slow cookers are versatile and can accommodate a wide variety of dishes such as soups, stews, meat seafood desserts and even beverages.

If you like this preview, then *click here for the full story of this eBook!*

Or go to: *http://www.amazon.com/dp/B00VUGNTYW/*

Check Out My Other Books

- *Chakras for Beginners: The Ultimate Guide to Balancing Chakras, Radiating Positive Energies and Strengthening Auras*
- *Anger, Stress and Fear: Your Personal Guide to Controlling Anger, Managing Stress and Overcoming Fear*
- *Ultimate Guide to Financial Freedom: Achieve Wealth, Attain Success and Manage Your Debt Like the Rich!*

Books of author Ricky King

- *10 Steps against Pornography: A Step Journey to Overcoming Internet Sexual Addiction through Jesus*
- *Gilgamesh: King in Quest of Immortality – An Extra-Biblical Proof for the Genesis Flood*
- *Israel vs. the World: The Apple of God's Eye in the End Times*

Books of author Tammi Diamond

- *Slimming Secrets: Health, Fitness, and Diet Secrets for the New You*
- *Gout Cure: Your Ultimate and Comprehensive Guide in Treating Gout Permanently*
- *Liver Cleanse and Detox Diet: The Ultimate Guide for Cleansing the Body, Eliminating Toxins and Losing Weight!*
- *10 Things You Need to Know about Ebola: Facts about the Virus, Symptoms, Quarantine and Prevention*
- *Anticancer Diet: The Ultimate Guide in Fighting Cancer, Lowering Cancer Risk and Achieving Optimum Health*
- *Pilates for Beginners: The Essential Guide to Total Body Fitness, Strong Muscles and Lean Body*

Dedication

To our three blessings that have made RicTamily complete and continue to grow together in His loving embrace.

Disclaimer

The information in this book is in no way intended as medical advice. This book is not meant to be used, nor should it be used, to diagnose or treat any medical condition. The author disclaims responsibility for any adverse health effects that come in combination with the use of methods and suggestions presented in the book. The publisher and author are not responsible for any health or allergy needs that may require medical supervision and are not liable for any damages or negative consequences from any treatment, action, application or preparation, to any person reading or following the information in this book.

www.ingramcontent.com/pod-product-compliance
Lightning Source LLC
Chambersburg PA
CBHW041151180526
45159CB00002BB/774